The Magic of Saffron

For Beauty and to Heal

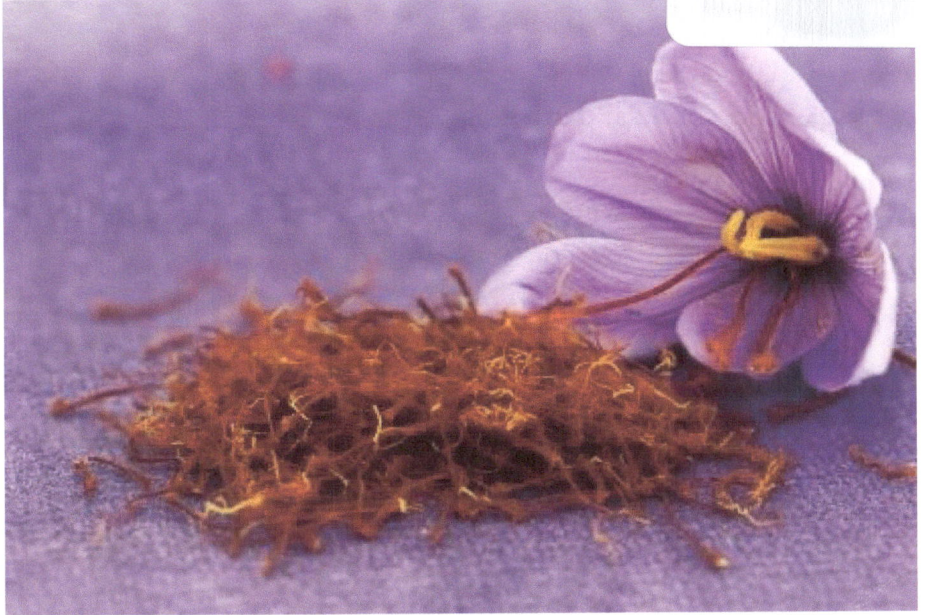

Health Learning Series

Dueep Jyot Singh

Mendon Cottage Books

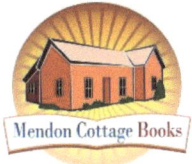

JD-Biz Publishing

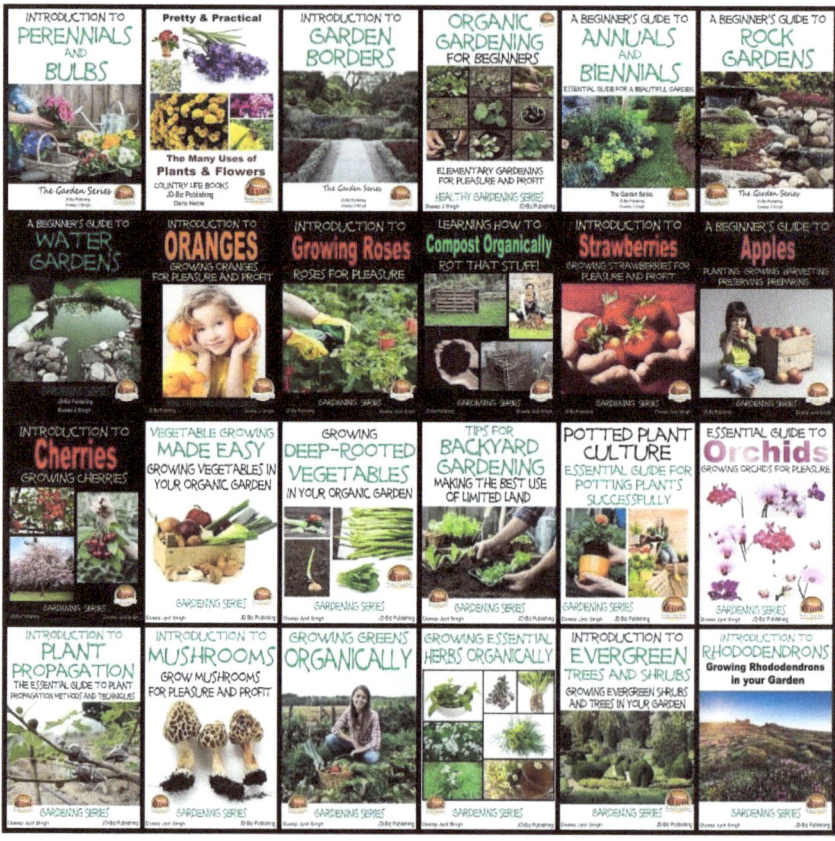

Our books are available at

1. Amazon.com
2. Barnes and Noble
3. Itunes
4. Kobo
5. Smashwords
6. Google Play Books

Table of Contents

Introduction

The moment you hear the word "saffron", your immediate reaction is the vision of an exotic, valuable and very expensive spice. You may also think of a golden – orangeish color.

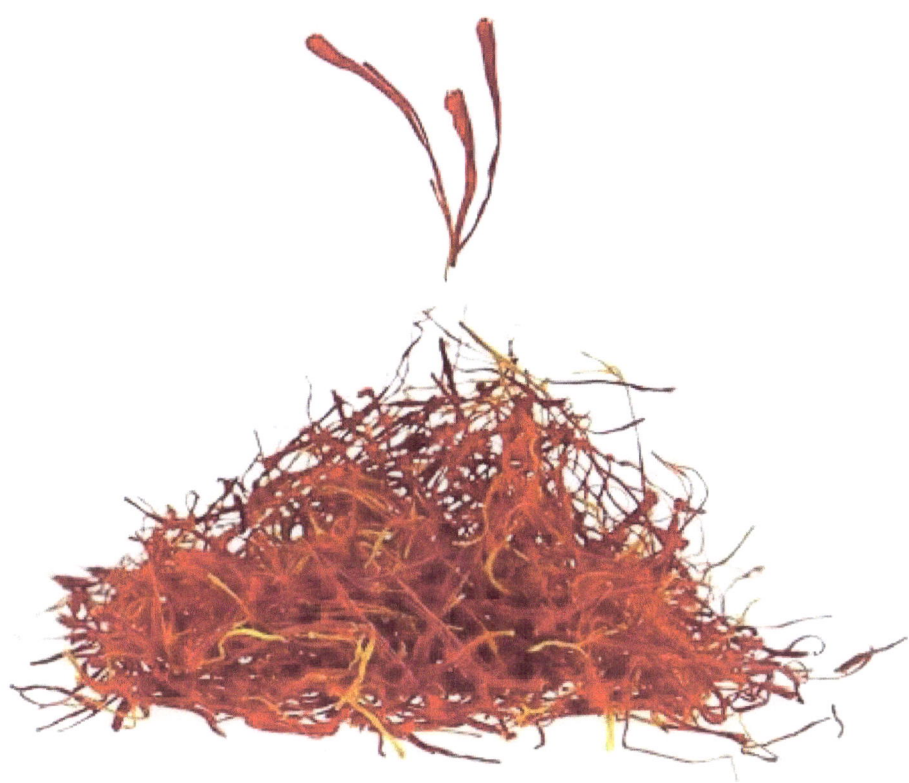

The term saffron comes from the Persian term Zaferan for orange gold. That is because the Persians were supposed to be the first of the culinary gourmets to use saffron in cooking. They already knew all about the healing qualities of this precious spice and used it extensively in medicine. But when they found out that just a couple of stigmas of the precious crocus was able to give their dishes a lovely tint, aroma, and look, saffron came into popular usage.

It is also said that saffron was used extensively in China, more than 2000 years ago, where it was used in herbal medicine. A saffron plant had up to four flowers. Each of them had three Crimson and bright stigmas. These stigmas are the most precious providers of saffron in their dried form.

In ancient Greece, which is also a contender for "we discovered saffron first," the people of Minoan and Cretan origin painted beautiful paintings of saffron collectors on their walls. Santorini excavations, going back to the Bronze Age, – more than 5000 years ago have extremely well defined frescoes of saffron collectors , wearing their native garb.[1]

This plant, belongs to the crocus family, and is called Crocus Sativus. It is supposed to be a native of Southwest Asia, from where it slowly and steadily spread to North America, North Africa, and Europe.

As time went by, and people began to use new sea routes to discover brave brand-new worlds, the demand for more and more saffron began to grow, especially in ancient civilizations where cuisine and the standard of living was steeped in luxury. This is why the conquering Romans who could not do without crocus, make sure that wherever they went, they did take some crocus bulbs and corms along with them. Since those long gone days, this is considered to be one of the most expensive and exotic of spices known to mankind.

Why is saffron so much in demand? In some Assyrian medicinal books going back to 7th-century BC, 90 illnesses were supposed to be cured with the use of saffron. Believe it or not, saffron based pigmentation dyes, used to dye clothing have been found in ancient Persia and Iran, going back to *50,000 years.* This was cultivated in the Isphahan,Darbena and Khorasan regions of Persia at that time. So I would not be surprised if this was one of the first spices to be cultivated by man, in his settlements along with garlic, onion, turmeric and other herbs.

Most of the saffron collected by the Sumerians and the Babylonians for their magic ceremonies were the stigmas of the wild crocus. Clothes with

---

[1] http://www.nmia.com/~jaybird/ThomasBakerPaintings/saffron_gatherer.html

saffron threads woven through them were offered up to the gods. Priests used to wear clothes, dyed rich golden red with saffron. The ordinary people just dyed their clothes with turmeric to get that same golden yellowish color.

It is said that Alexander the Great was rather envious of the quality of the saffron grown in Persia, that he demanded that a major portion of it be allotted to his own personal use and for the use of his soldiers in order to heal their wounds.

This was done by making a paste of milk, honey and saffron and applying it on the wounds. I am sure it was the honey which cured the infections and aided in the healing process. But the idea of taking a luxurious bath in saffron tinted water became part of the Greek lifestyle after Alexander conquered Persia.

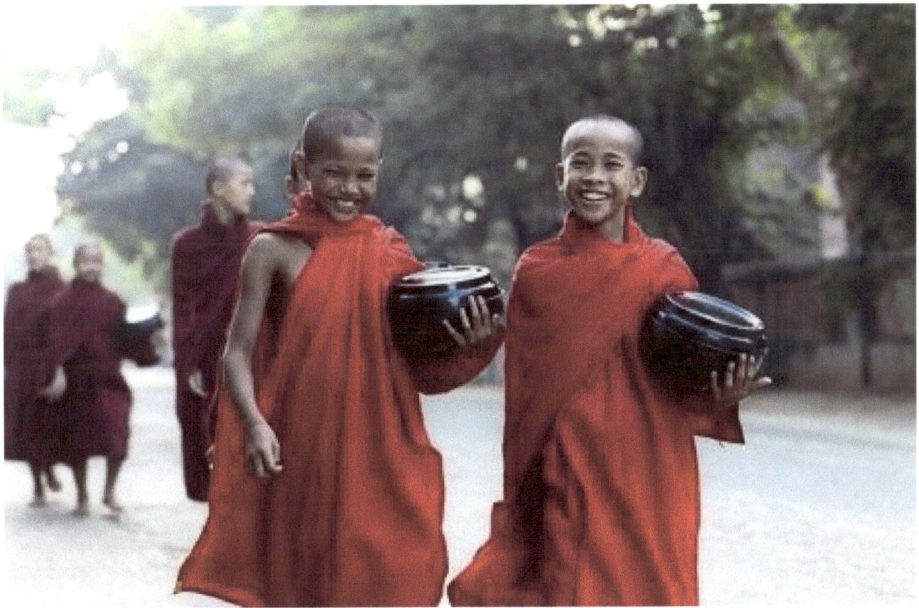

Traditional robes of monks were dyed in saffron, since ancient times. Nowadays, other natural dyes are used to give the rich color.

According to Chinese history, Kashmir was the place where saffron grew in abundance in ancient times. Travelers and traders from all over the world came to Kashmir to get this precious saffron, which was used as a cure for melancholia and as a golden color tint and dye. The local Kashmiris dyed their clothes with saffron, turmeric, gamboge and jackfruit for that particular golden red color, depending on the availability of the available spice, vegetable or herb.

Saffron is cultivated in Pennsylvania, having been brought there by the Dutch in the 18th century from Europe. Lancaster County growers still grow saffron from corms brought from Europe by their forefathers to America.

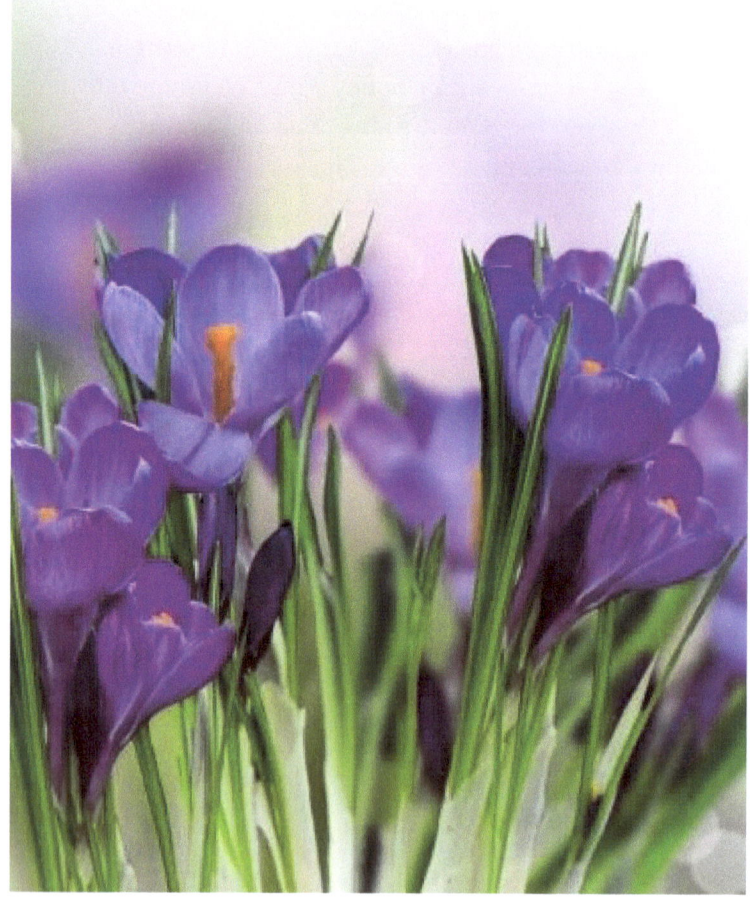

Saffron has also been the cause of wars. In the 14th century, when the Black Death had Europe in its grip, saffron was considered to be the only curative and preventive medicine. So this precious thread was shipped from Italy and Spain through Genoa and other Mediterranean ports like Rhodes. So pirates

– who incidentally happen to be noblemen – began to prey on these ships, thus causing A Saffron War, which lasted for 14 weeks.

The fear of such occurrences happening again made people start cultivating saffron in Germany – Nuremberg and in Basel. They also had a law be said that anybody found adulterating saffron would immediately be imprisoned, and executed.

But even so, saffron continued to be adulterated. To this day, you cannot be quite sure that the very excellent strands of saffron that you are buying are the real thing or not. It could have been adulterated with other dried stigmas , or steeped in honey in order to increase the weight. They were also mixed with silk fibers dyed orange.

So this is how you recognize pure saffron.

Saffron Test

Take a strand of saffron and put it in your mouth. Real saffron is immediately going to give you a feeling of "heat" and is going to taste bitter.

After that, you are going to put the strands in water. Leave it for a little while and then soak a piece of white cloth in the water. Upon rubbing, you should see an immediate saffron red stain of true saffron. If you see a red stain which turns yellow, afterwards, that means the saffron has been adulterated.

Pharmacists normally use rectified spirit in order to check the purity of saffron. They put a little bit of saffron in a little bit of Spirit, and see whether the spirit turns orange in color or not. Also, the color of the stigmas should not change when it comes in contact with the Spirit.

How to Use Saffron?

Traditionally, it is normally bruised gently in a pestle and mortar with a little bit of milk. You can also steep it in a little bit of milk before you add it for tinting purposes to any dish. Apart from its medical value, it is going to impart a golden color, as well as rich flavor to sweetmeats, rice and other dishes.

Cultivating Saffron

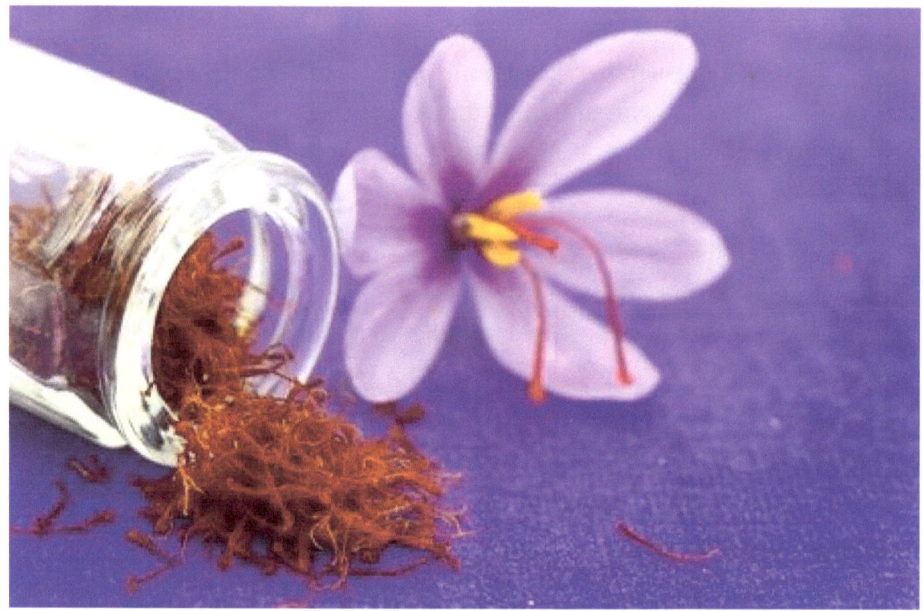

If you are under the impression that growing red gold is difficult, do not worry. That is not so. The only problem is that harvesting saffron comes rather expensive, so if you are living in an area where labor comes high, well, saffron growing can just be an interesting hobby.

Remember, that 150 flowers are going to give you 1 g of saffron and a saffron plant has two – four flowers. So do the math, when you are planting the corms.

Saffron can be grown anywhere in the world. That is why it is grown extensively places where labor is cheap and the soil rich and nutritious.

Saffron corm planting is normally done from June until the middle of September. It is going to start flowering from the month of October, a year from the time it has been planted.

The winter is normally used productively by the plant for extensive vegetative development. Do not worry if the leaves dry out in the summer. They are going to come up again in time for flowering.

Right Soil for Saffron

Saffron does not bother much about the climate; rather, your priority has to be the soil. The soil should be well drained. Do not use heavy clay soil.

The best soil is, of course, one of a pH value 6 – 8. This is the neutral soil with plenty of silt or is calcareous with just a little bit of clay.

I would suggest growing this plant, just for fun in your garden as a simple border or in your vegetable garden in soil which has been improved by adding garden compost, peat and sand.

Saffron loves the sun, so make sure that you plant it where there is plenty of sunshine, especially in the autumn, when it is going to burst out in full bloom.

Preparation of the Soil

Soil preparation is really necessary to get the full benefit of a rich harvest.

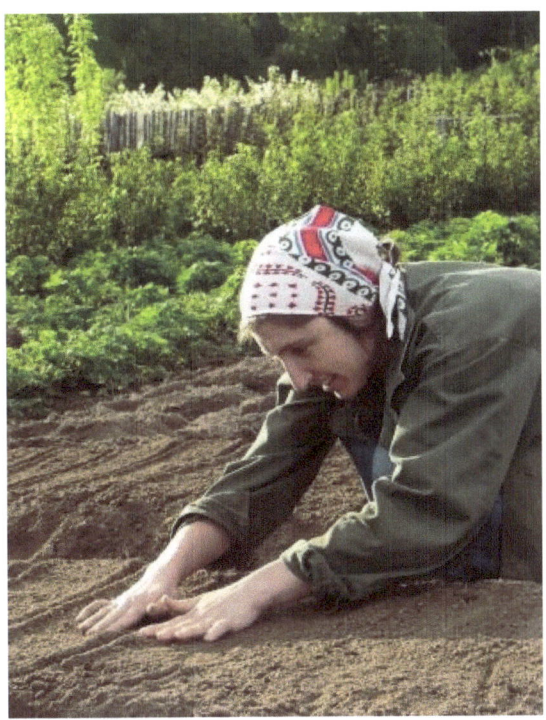

Just the feel of well turned over soil – plowed to 20 cm and mixed with organic garden compost or green manure – can be such a rejuvenating feeling!

If you are using any sort of natural fertilizer, which has nitrogen in it, spread it all over the soil surface after you have planted the corms.

Crocus bulbs/corms are available in nurseries all over the world. Ask for Crocus Sativus. This is the original true saffron plant.

The ground is of course going to be totally free of weeds. Loosen the soil a little, with a little bit of hoeing, before you begin to plant the corms.You can plan these corms, either directly into the ground, outside or inside the window boxes or any other sort of containers.

These corms are going to be planted at a depth of 10 – 15 cm. [Up to 6 inches.]. Leave a space of about 4 to 5 inches between the corms.Just use enough of water to keep the soil moist. Do not overwater, especially during the summer.

This is a perennial plant, so one corm is going to multiply into about five corms in about three years.

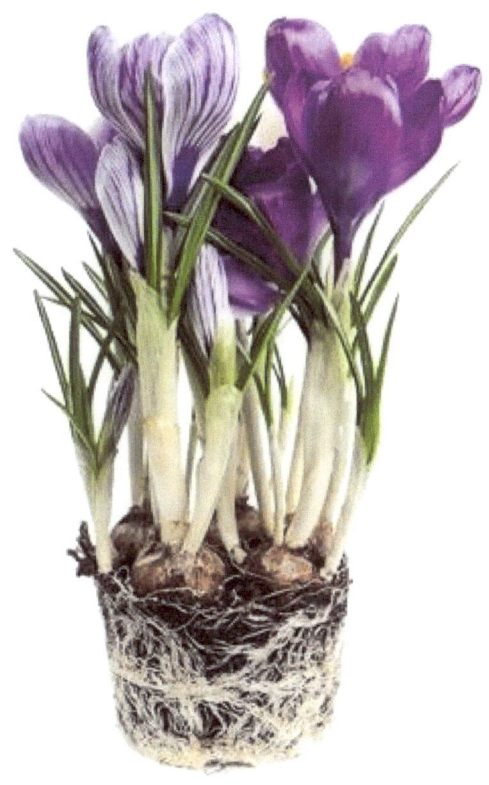

Crocus Diseases and Infections

Just like other plants, saffron is also very vulnerable to fungal infections, as well as viruses and bacteria. Brown ulceration is caused by Rhizoctonia crocorum which is a fungus like Fusarium which attacks the leaves and the corm.

Plenty of damp is going to cause damp rot which is also known as Violet Root Rot. This is contagious and farmers are very worried about it, destroying huge harvests. As prevention is better than cure, this can be prevented by making sure that the plants are not planted in a muggy and moist atmosphere and waterlogged soil.

These diseases normally appear after around three years. So I would suggest preventing them by digging up the corms, if your field is infected, and plant them again in another field. Traditionally, the productive capacity of a saffron bearing field should not be more than 10 years.

Harvesting Your Saffron

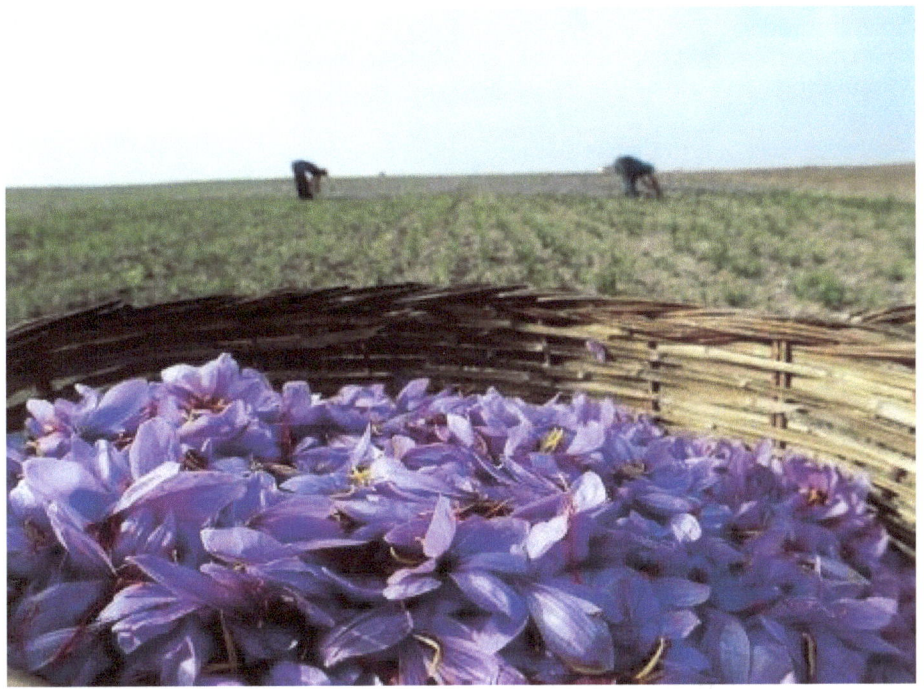

Saffron normally starts blooming in October, during the first year. It is going to last for a month, up to November.

Traditionally, harvesting was done by hand by the whole village which used to wake up at dawn on the days flowers bloomed in October. Then they would wait for the sunrise and the flower to open. Dawn harvesting was done traditionally because the flower began to wilt away with the passing of the day.

These flowers were picked by hand. If you have a small number of flowers to pick, just leave the flower on, and pick the three red and precious stigmas – filaments with a pair of tweezers.

This is a modern innovation and is known as trimming.

However, if you are picking in large quantities and are strapped for time, pick all the flowers and leave the stigmas to be picked up by another group simultaneously. This was normally done with another group sitting around a table, singing and gossiping, while their hands picked the stigmas busily.

That is because it is easier to trim the freshly harvested flowers and get the stigmas picked with tweezers, scissors, or even with one's nails.

And then, later on in the week there would be a feast given by the farmyard owner/landlord after the harvest had been gathered in because another precious crop of saffron had come through all its ensuing perils like mice, insects, fungus, possible rain, etc. to rich harvest.

The purple petals and the other stigmas which are yellow in color are gathered and put into the garden in the compost heap.

Drying of Saffron

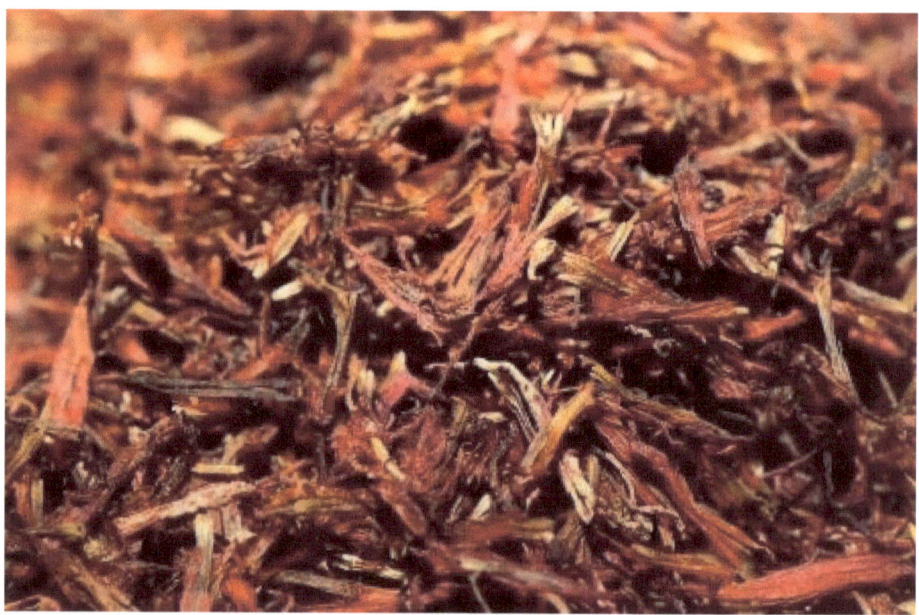

You need to dry these filaments before you can put them to use. This was done traditionally by putting the stigmas in large sieves and placing them in the sun. The temperature was around 40 – 60°C. You can also dry them out in your oven, leaving the door open slightly.

The stigmas are going to be really breakable after they have been dried completely. They are also going to be very light. You will need to store them immediately in an airtight container, and place them in a cool and dry spot in your kitchen.

Traditionally, Saffron, which has been stored away is left to age for about a month, before it is put to use. Two years is the age limit for saffron.

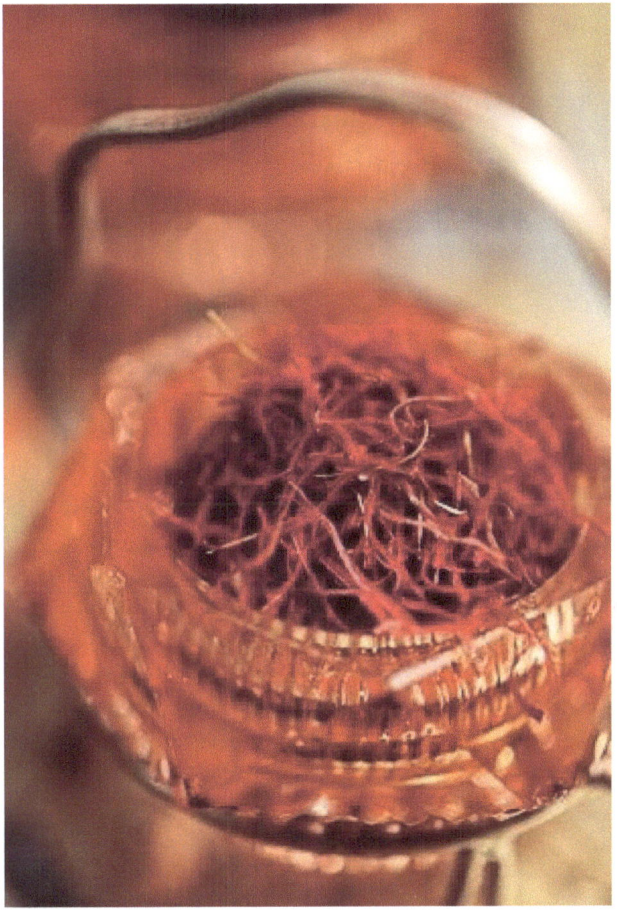

So what is the yield that you are going to get? In the first year, you are going to get one flower from about 70% of the corms. In the second and third year, you may get about two flowers per corm, but they are multiplying underneath. If you are lucky, you may get up to four flowers per corm in the third year and beyond.

You can divide the corms, after digging them up and then replanting them. That means, one corm, which has survived one season is capable of giving you 10 cormlets in this vegetative method of propagation. As saffron is incapable of producing any sort of seeds, this is the only way in which you can grow it.

You are going to get a plant growing up to a height of up to 12 inches with about 4 – 11 white leaves which are non-photosynthetic. These are going to cover the true leaves of the crocus, while they are developing and budding.

The flower is purple in color and is going to appear in October. The fragrance of the crocus, which is light and honey like, is considered to be very intoxicating especially where this flower is grown in large quantities.

No wonder this was grown extensively in the Mediterranean region where the dry and the hot summer like in the Mediterranean Maquis and the American and Spanish chaparral are conducive to an excellent harvest of Crocus Sativus. So if you are living in an area, where the climate is dry, but you can get plenty of spring rain and dry summers, start growing crocus there. Cold weather and plenty of rainy weather in October is going to give you diseased plants, and a low harvest.

If you get rain just before the flowers are about to bloom, you are going to get an excellent harvest. That is why the yields of harvests in Greece, Spain, and Kashmir give the best quality of saffron.

Crocuses enjoy plenty of sun, but they do not flourish in the shade. Full sunlight is necessary for their growth, especially on slopes where you can get direct sunlight. The quality of the ensuing saffron is going to be higher, if you plant the mother corm really deeply – up to 6 inches deep in Morocco, Spain, and in Greece.

You can boost up the productivity of your crocus field, by providing it with lots of organic manure. Traditionally, 30 tons of manure was given to the land per hectare to feed the crocuses, before planting the corms. Nowadays, you can just sprinkle the manure on top of the soil, after you have planted and watered your field.

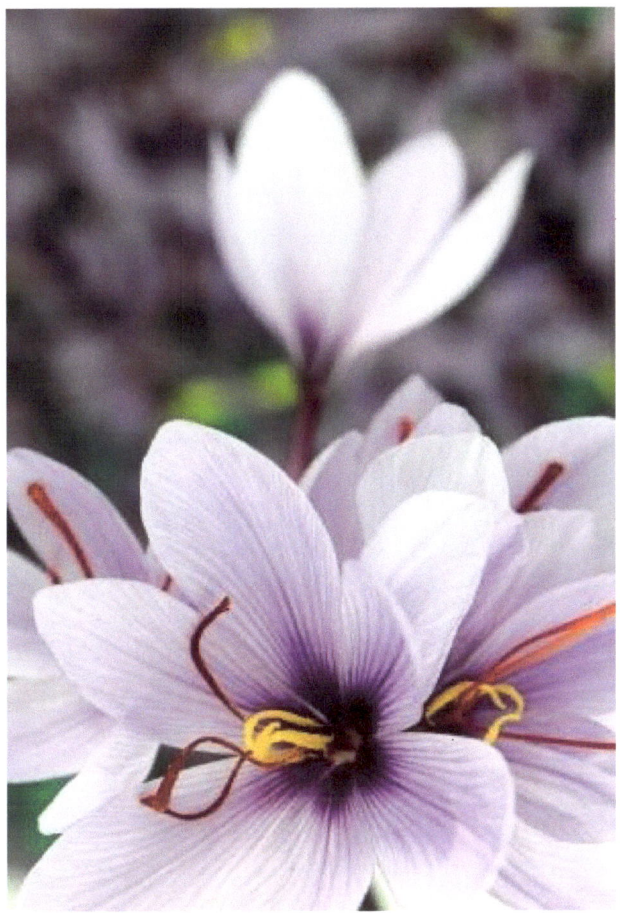

Iran produces about 90% of the world's saffron. After that comes Greece, which produces 5.7 tons per year, followed by Morocco and Kashmir. The world's output is 300 tons of filament and powder. 1 pound – 450 g of dried saffron is going to be obtained by harvesting 75,000 flowers. 150, 000 flowers or 1 kg of precious saffron can be obtained through more than 40 hours of picking and labor. That is why they retail for around USD17 for about .06 ounces.

Fresh saffron is going to be slightly moist, elastic, vivid crimson in color and without any broken thread debris.

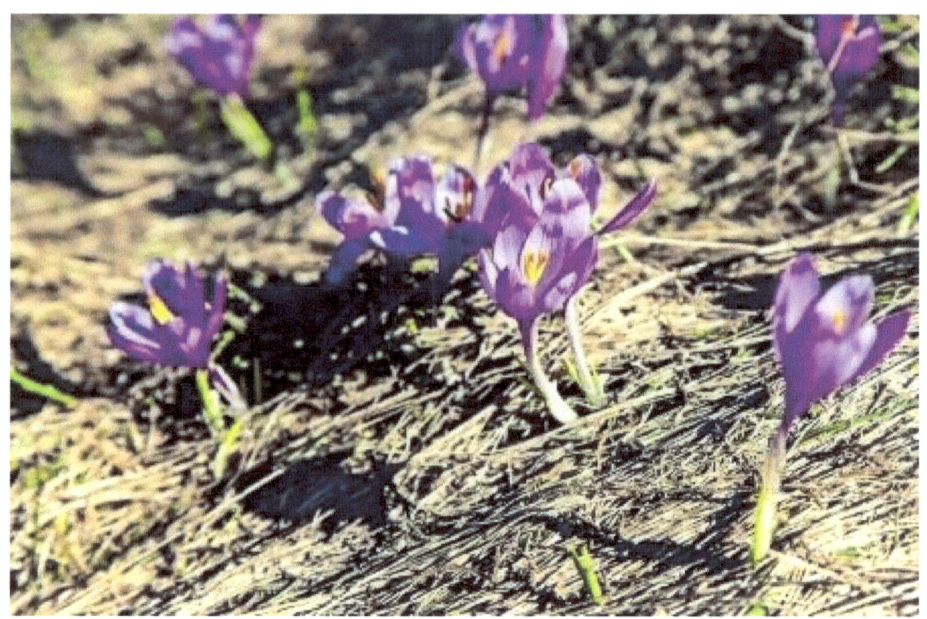

Using Saffron in Cuisine

A few filaments of saffron are bruised and then soaked for about 10 minutes in hot water before you intend to use them. This is going to release all the natural components present in them. Traditional usage down the ages in various cuisines have been to color Italian risotto, Spanish paella , Persian pulavs and naturally biryanis.

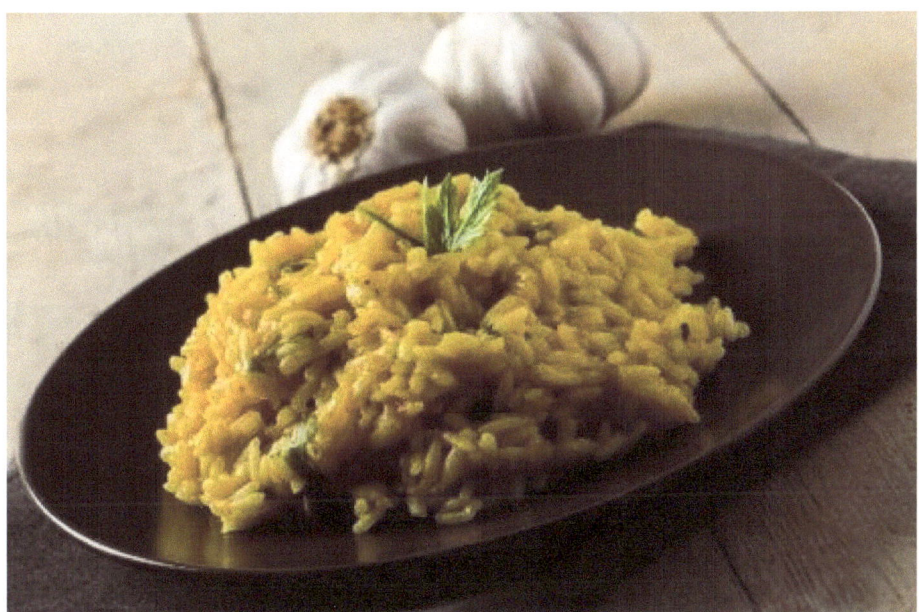

Saffron Tinted Risotto

Saffron is considered to have a warming "Constitution". That is why it is eaten more in winter.

3.5 ounces of saffron or hundred grams is going to have 310 kcal, 11.43 g of protein and a number of vitamins, including vitamin A, Riboflavin, calcium, phosphorous, magnesium, iron, sodium and potassium.

Traditional Cooling Saffron – Almond Drink

This drink is normally prepared in the summer, and drunk in large amounts to cool down your system, especially when it is 30° plus outside. You can adjust the amounts according to how much you want to drink of this healthy milk-based drink. This is what is normally served to guests in the summer, in the Indian subcontinent when you do not have fresh lemon juice around.

I am giving you the amount for 25 – 30 glasses, so that you can just make it and put it in the fridge. The spices used here are used in less quantities, because after all it is the summer, and you want a refreshing healthy drink.

2 L of milk, 1 L of water, 25 almonds, 4 small green cardamoms, 1 inch piece of cinnamon, a few strands of saffron, eight black peppercorns, 30 green pistachios, 20 cashew nuts, 3 tablespoons full of poppy seeds and 1 cup of sugar, or as per taste.

Soak the poppy seeds in cold water for 30 minutes before you grind them.

Dip the almonds in warm water for 10 minutes. You can now peel off the skin easily.

Boil the milk and add sugar. Now add the saffron strands to the hot milk. Put the milk in the refrigerator after it has cooled down a little so that it starts to chill.

Now grind the green cardamoms, cinema, and peppercorns to a fine powder.

Grind the almonds, pistachios, cashew nuts, and poppy seeds with a little bit of milk, so that you get a finely ground paste. Mix the powder and the paste together and then add to the chilled milk. Blend well.

Either put it back into the fridge for more chilling, or serve immediately. Traditionally, a little bit of rosewater or vanilla water is sprinkled on this coolant.

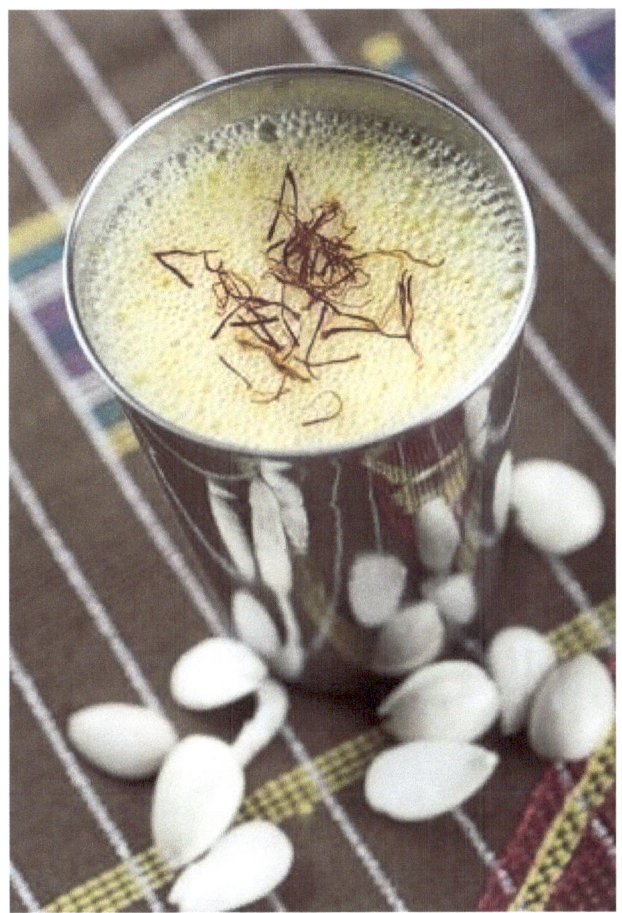

This is known as Thandai (Thunn- daaee) or literally, "Coolant"

Saffron for Beauty and Health

Saffron for Lightening the Complexion

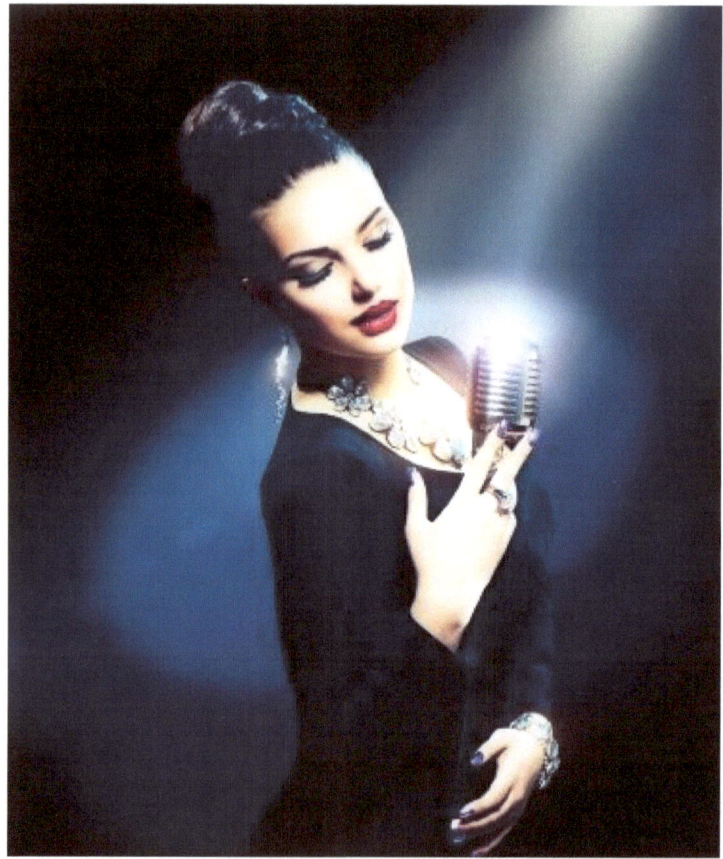

Monday's child is fair of face…

Saffron was considered to be one of the greatest and most beneficial of beauty aids, by all the ancient beauties, including Cleopatra. She used saffron lotions and saffron baths in order to keep young and youthful.

Here is a traditional beauty remedy, which was passed on to me by a friend, who was dusky in complexion. Her grandmother had told her this remedy, which was supposed to lighten the complexion and make it fair.

Beauty lotion

Take 250 g of milk. Now add five filaments of saffron to it along with one small cardamom. Drink this milk every day, and find your complexion growing fairer and lovelier. Ancient beauties in these swore by this health beauty drink. They drank it for one month in the winters, and the long-term cumulative affect lasted till the next winter when they repeated it again.

Use just that much of saffron, which tints the color of the milk. Do not overdo the saffron, because after all it is a powerful spice in its own right.

Saffron to Cure Diseases

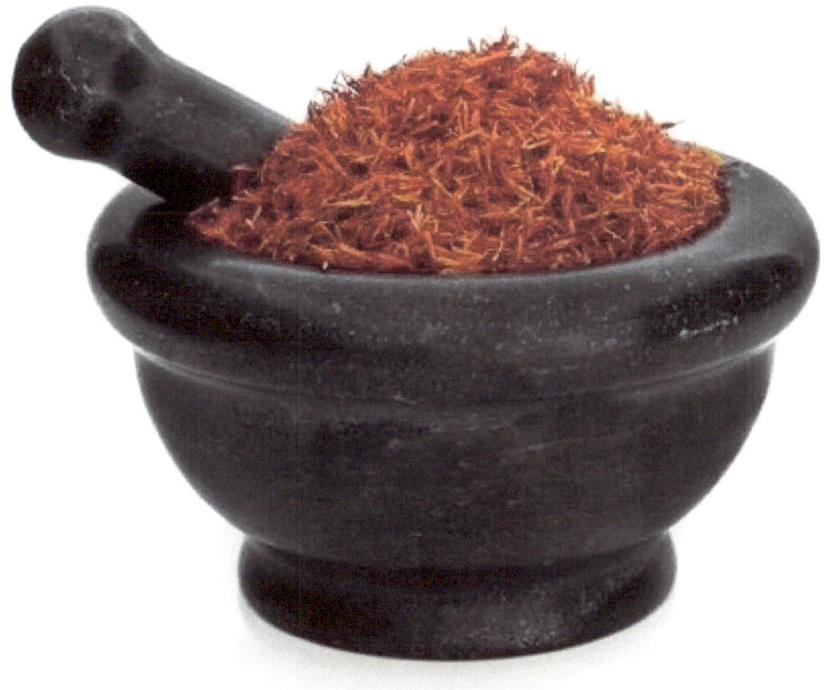

Depression Cure

Saffron has been used to cure hysteria as well as depression, for ages. The Romans knew about it. So did the Chinese! Women suffering from hysteria were given saffron. It is only modern research, which has proven that saffron has elements which enhance the production of mood enhancing neurotransmitters like Dopamine and norepinephrine, which is normally secreted by the body, the moment you get stressed out, or tense.

Researchers have proven that 30 mg of saffron taken regularly for six weeks has given positive results in depression. No anti-depressants were given during this time. So does this not prove that natural remedies are the equivalent of chemical drugs, and can manage to cure you, naturally, without harmful side effects.

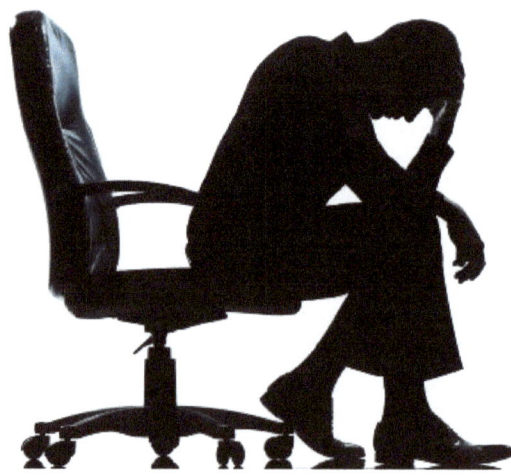

Feeling depressed? Saffron has been used down the ages to cure depression and to reduce stress and tension. Drink 30 mg of saffron, [13 filaments] in a glass of warm milk, every night before going to sleep.

Getting Rid of Kidney Stones

Any sort of uric acid stones in your body, can be eliminated with the regular use of six filaments of saffron in 1 cup of fresh grape juice. Keep drinking this until you get totally cured and the stones are eliminated altogether.

Saffron as a Cold Preventative and Cure

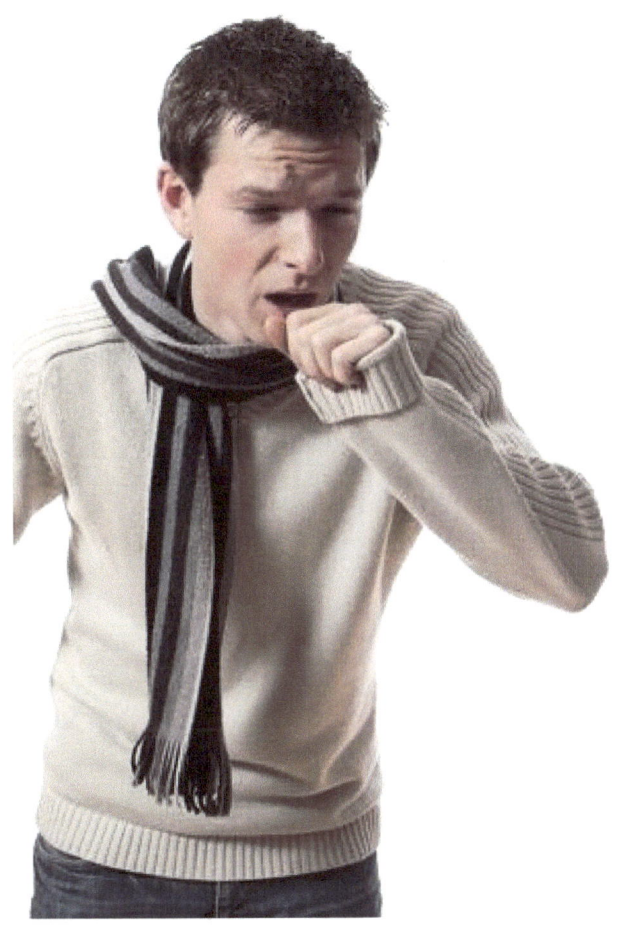

Saffron is excellent as the warming remedy during cold weather. Drink saffron milk to boost up your immunity system and to prevent yourself suffering from fever, cough, cold and other cold associated problems. You are going to drink this morning and night. This strengthens the respiratory system. It also regulates low blood pressure and gives you strength.

Saffron Milk

You are going to take a glass of warm milk and add five filaments of saffron to it. Drink this when you are ready to go to bed. The saffron is going to dissolve in the milk, especially if you have powdered the filaments beforehand.

Saffron as a Headache Remedy

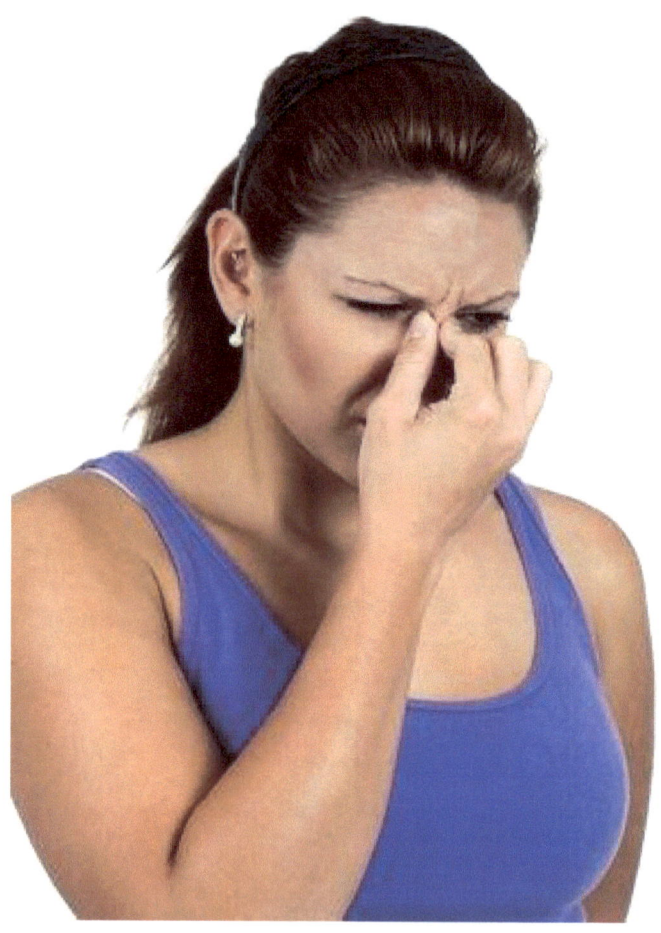

If I lived in olden times – Babylonian, Roman, Egyptian, Phoenician, Minoan, Cretan – and suffered from a headache, it is possible that my favorite slave would have massaged a paste of saffron on my forehead. Another of these slaveys would have placed some saffron – maybe 4 strands – in a little milk on a silver platter, and swirled it in front of my nose until I could be restored enough to get up and have a saffron bath to prepare myself for the evenings' festivities.

But I live in the 21st century, and I do not have any slaveys nor do I have silver platters. So I just mix the milk and the saffron in any sort of small container, which I can swing to and fro under my prominent proboscis and inhale.

I would not be surprised that the deep inhalation of this beautiful fragrance auto suggests my mind to get rid of the headache and fast!

But rubbing this mixture on the forehead was the traditional way of getting rid of migraines. You may want to try it out, if you suffer from these terribly painful and debilitating headaches which leave you all wrung out and helpless. [2]You can also sip saffron milk – with honey instead of sugar added to it – to get rid of the stress which may have caused that tension headache and migraine.

---

[2] Been There, Seen That ad nauseam no pun intended.

Best Moisturizing Lotion

Soak five filaments of saffron in milk overnight. The next morning, dip a ball of cotton in this and wipe your face, neck, and exposed areas of the skin. Leave on for half an hour before you wash it off with warm water.

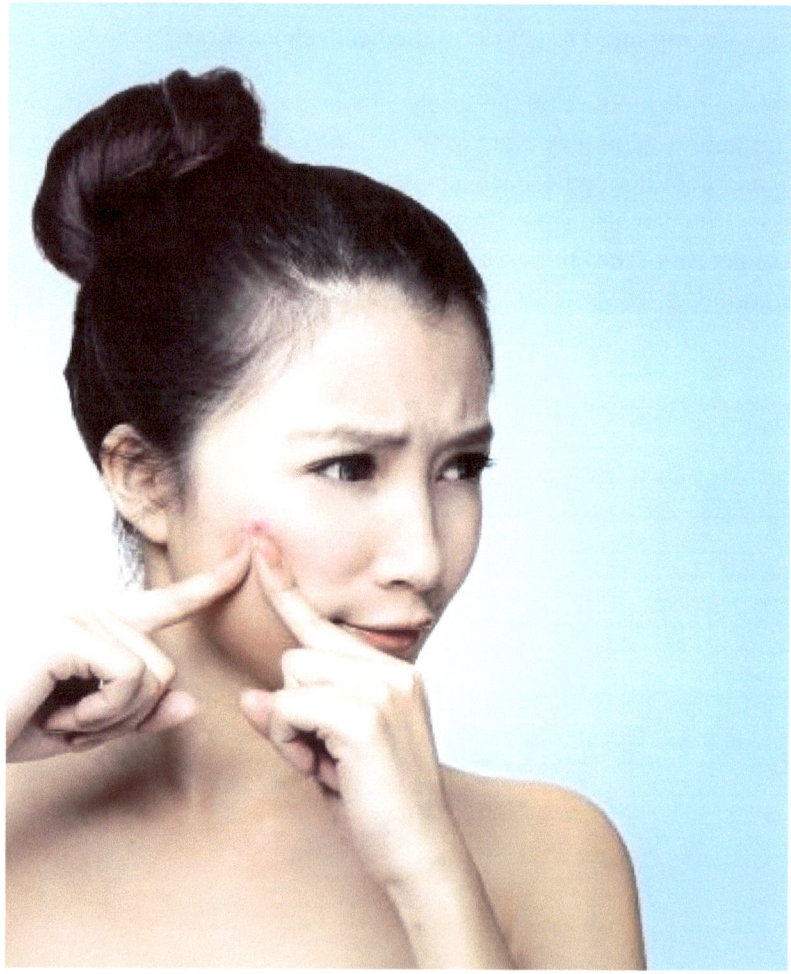

Pressing or fiddling with pimples is going to cause the infection to grow. Instead, keep your skin well moisturized and clean with a milk saffron lotion/moisturizer.

Try this treatment for about a month and look at the difference in the texture of your skin and the glow which has appeared. It is also an excellent way in which you can get rid of pimples.

In many parts of the East, fair is beautiful and the standard for desirability, especially in eligible young maidens, getting ready for marriage. Is it a surprise that an expectant mother drank saffron milk, so that her offspring – male or female – would be fair in complexion?

Thinking of it, I consider this rather a foolish procedure, because if you are genetically dark complexioned, you cannot have really fair offspring unless of course the mother chose a partner who was many tones "fairer" than her. And this was done often in ancient times in the East. And the mother used to pass off the offspring, with a much lighter skin tone as being the product of saffron milk!

Saffron for Women's Personal Health

Also, they could get rid of an unwanted pregnancy without anybody knowing about it by eating saffron in large quantities, over a large period of time. That would cause a natural miscarriage due to the "heat" produced by the saffron, which is a powerful "heat producing" spice, like cloves, cardamoms and cinnamon.

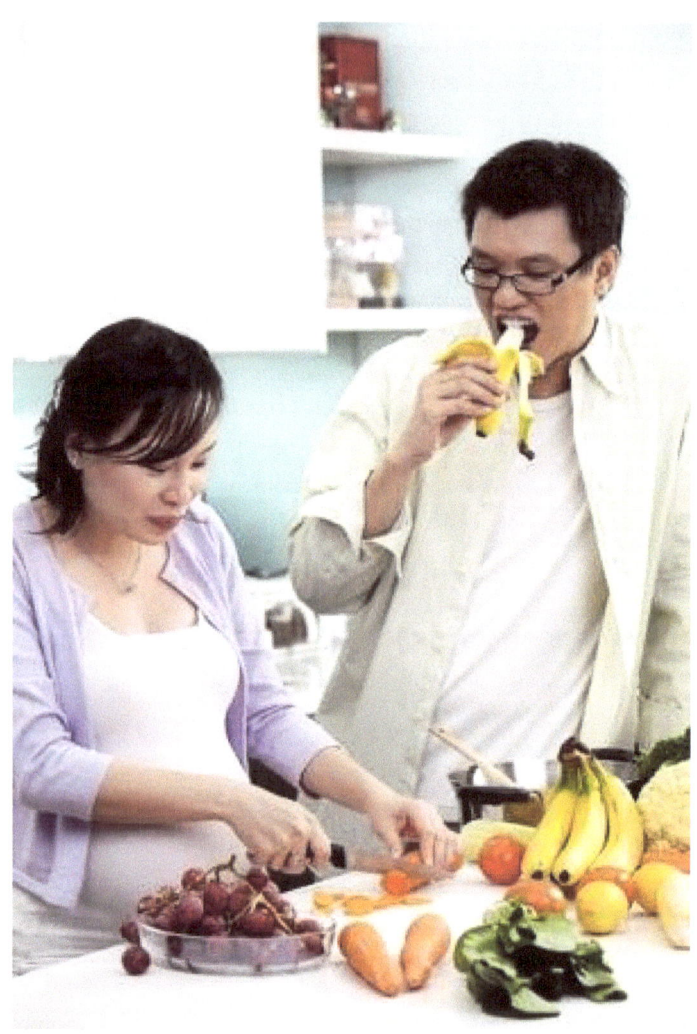

Apart from a healthy food/fruit diet, mom can be sure of a healthy baby by drinking lots of milk. Put three filaments of saffron in your milk drink, once every three days. That should be enough. We do not want to overdo it, do we! And baby is going to be fairer in complexion than mama and papa! So say they, in the East!

Also, a woman going through labor was traditionally given a cup of hot tea with some saffron strands added to it. This reduced the intensity of the pain and facilitated the birthing trauma for both mother and child.

My grandmother recounts that a newborn child was given a "lick" of honey mixed with saffron, as the first "meal" before taken to the mother for the first feed. In fact, my brand-new grandfather gave it to me, because that is ancient tradition in the East. It also prevented the child from suffering from infection, especially in a possibly unhealthy atmosphere of a stuffy ill ventilated room, and unhygienic surroundings.

Nevertheless, even today, saffron milk is drunk to cure what is coyly known as "women's problems."Women suffering from problems in the uterus could get rid of it through a regular use of saffron milk.

 Stomach cramps, especially during "those days" could be regulated with the use of saffron. So if you are suffering from this particular problem, all you have to do is take five strands of saffron and just a very very little bit of **edible camphor**.

Drink this mixture two times a day, beginning four days before you expect your monthly flow. Not only is it going to regulate the flow, but it is also going to prevent and cure stomach cramps.

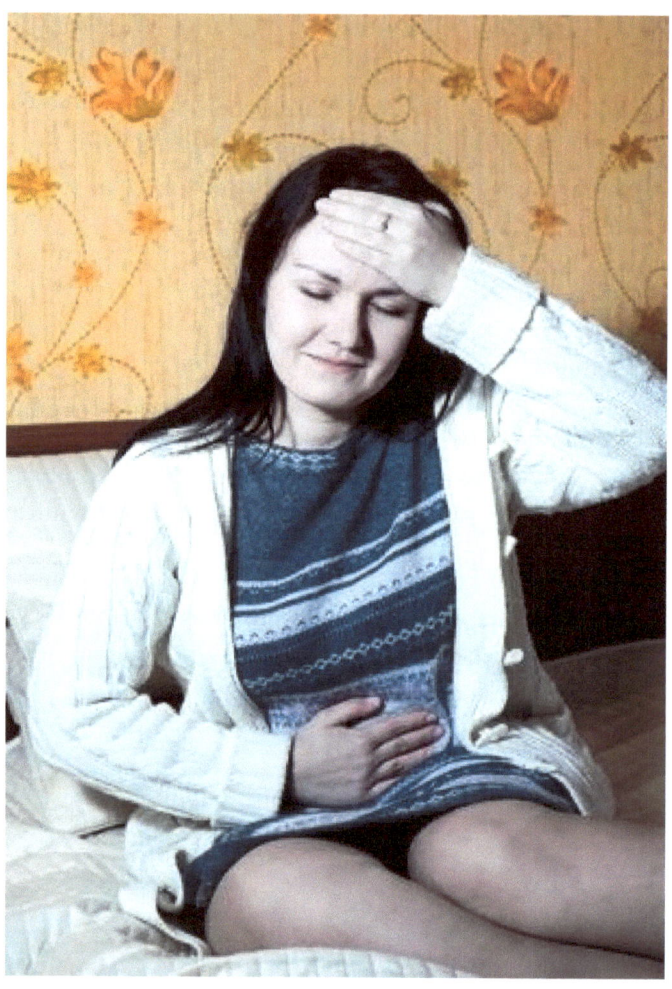

Looks like tummy problems and a possibly feverish head ailment here. Use a saffron milk paste on the forehead and drink saffron milk to prevent a possible infection and to heal you from inside by boosting up your immunity system and by fighting the bacteria/viruses.

Teething problems

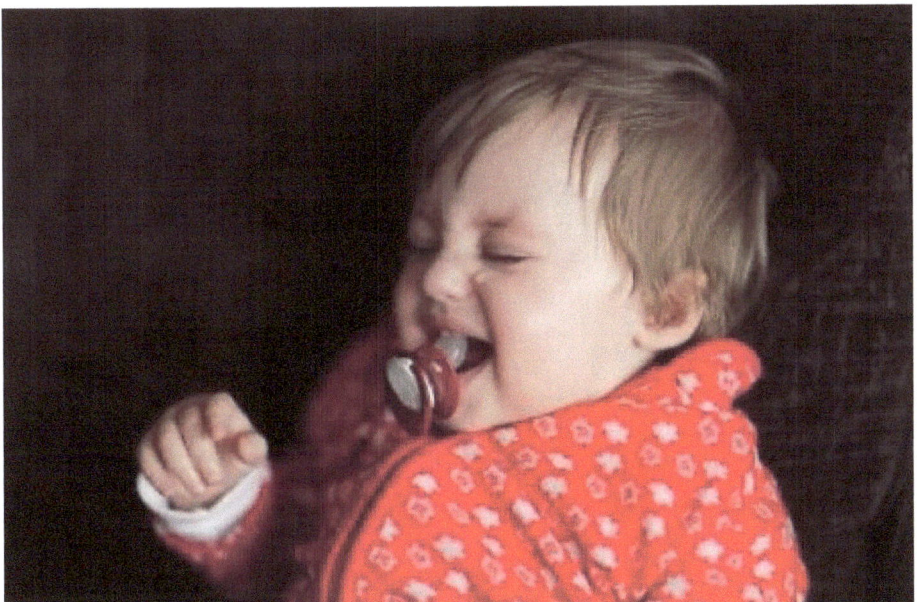

Infants suffering from teething problems can be given three filaments of saffron in milk and honey. They are not going to make such a feverish fuss because they are going to be getting plenty of vitamin B and riboflavin, as well as the lessening of pain, thanks to the honey and saffron.

Appendix

Where Do You Get Edible Camphor?

There are two types of camphor available in the market today. One is the chemically prepared camphor, which is normally used in religious ceremonies, to give out a sweet aroma, when burned as an incense before the deities. Do not eat chemically prepared camphor.

I have been trying to find edible camphor in my area without much luck, except for in one 75-year-old shop, and he was out of the real stuff. But it is supposedly available in parts of South India under the name of "Paccha karpooram."

200 g of this original edible stuff is for around USD10 from this seller – http://www.cosmosdelhi.com/products/edible-camphor---pacha-karpooram/pages/all-products

You may also want to read about the beneficial qualities of edible, as well as ordinary camphor in this news article.

http://www.newindianexpress.com/lifestyle/health/article1350482.ece

Remember, that it is considered to be dangerous when you ingest it in large quantities. That is because you are not eating the edible product.

But if it helps get rid of the painful cramps, and regulates your monthly flow, without resort to any sort of powerful drugs, possibly you will think it well worth keeping in your medicine cabinet.

Conclusion

This book has introduced to the magic of Saffron. So start adding it to your cuisine, look for Crocus Sativus corms to grow in your garden, and use it for healing like the ancients did. Thus you can enjoy the wisdom of the ages.

Live Long and Prosper!

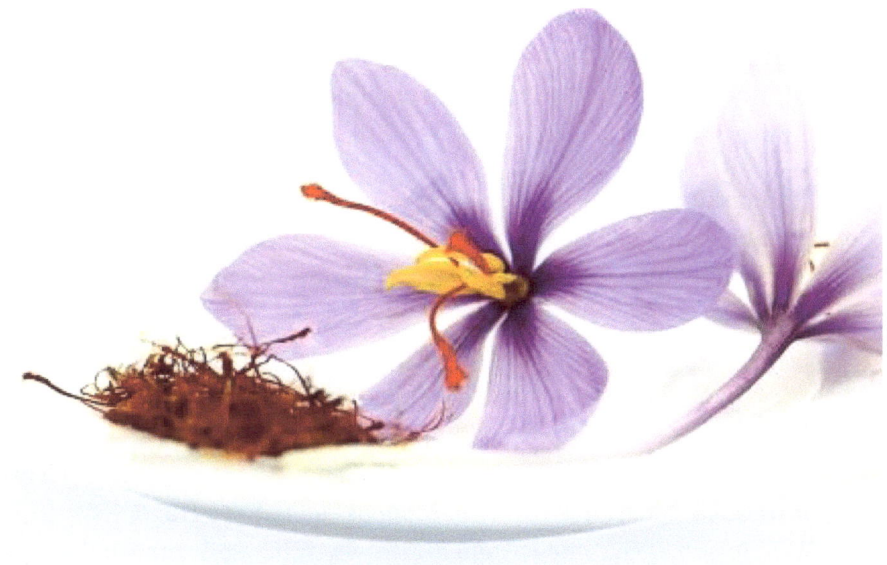

Author Bio

Dueep Jyot Singh is a Management and IT Professional who managed to gather Postgraduate qualifications in Management and English and Degrees in Science, French and Education while pursuing different enjoyable career options like being an hospital administrator, IT,SEO and HRD Database Manager/ trainer, movie , radio and TV scriptwriter, theatre artiste and public speaker, lecturer in French, Marketing and Advertising, ex-Editor of Hearts On Fire (now known as Solstice) Books Missouri USA, advice columnist and cartoonist, publisher and Aviation School trainer, ex-moderator on Medico.in, banker, student councilor ,travelogue writer … among other things!

One fine morning, she decided that she had enough of killing herself by Degrees and went back to her first love -- writing. It's more enjoyable! She already has 48 published academic and 14 fiction- in- different- genre books under her belt.

When she is not designing websites or making Graphic design illustrations for clients , she is browsing through old bookshops hunting for treasures, of which she has an enviable collection – including R.L. Stevenson, O.Henry, Dornford Yates, Maurice Walsh, De Maupassant, Victor Hugo, Sapper, C.N. Williamson, "Bartimeus" and the crown of her collection- Dickens "The Old Curiosity Shop," and so on… Just call her "Renaissance Woman") - collecting herbal remedies, acting like Universal Helping Hand/Agony Aunt, or escaping to her dear mountains for a bit of exploring, collecting herbs and plants and trekking.

Check out some of the other JD-Biz Publishing books

Gardening Series on Amazon

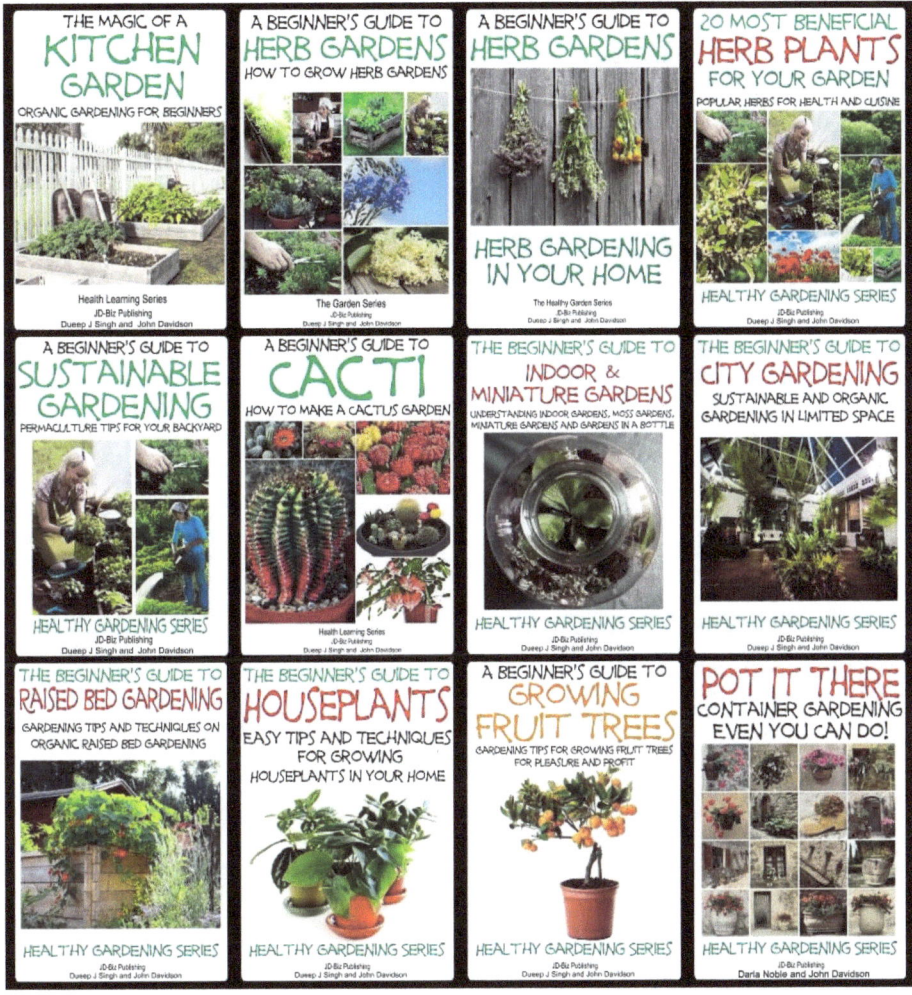

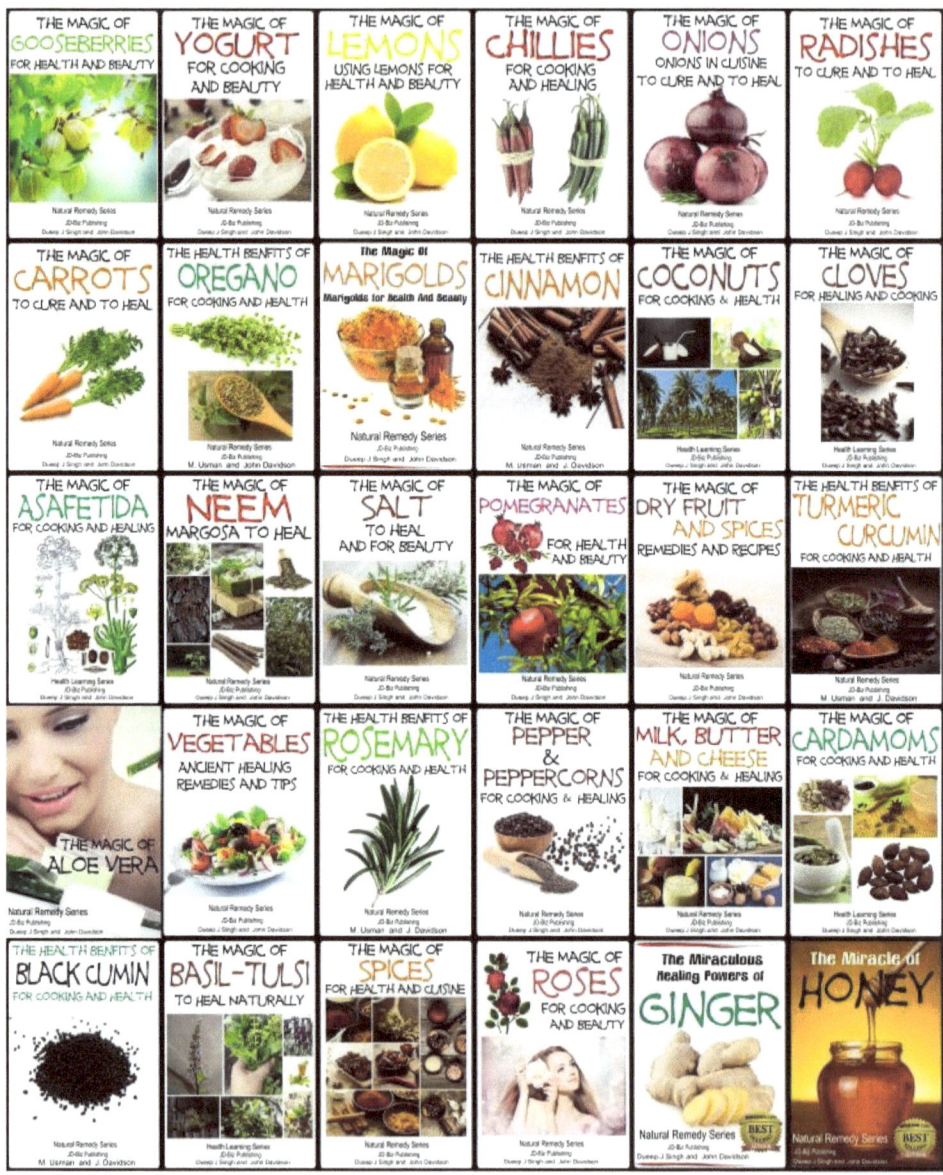

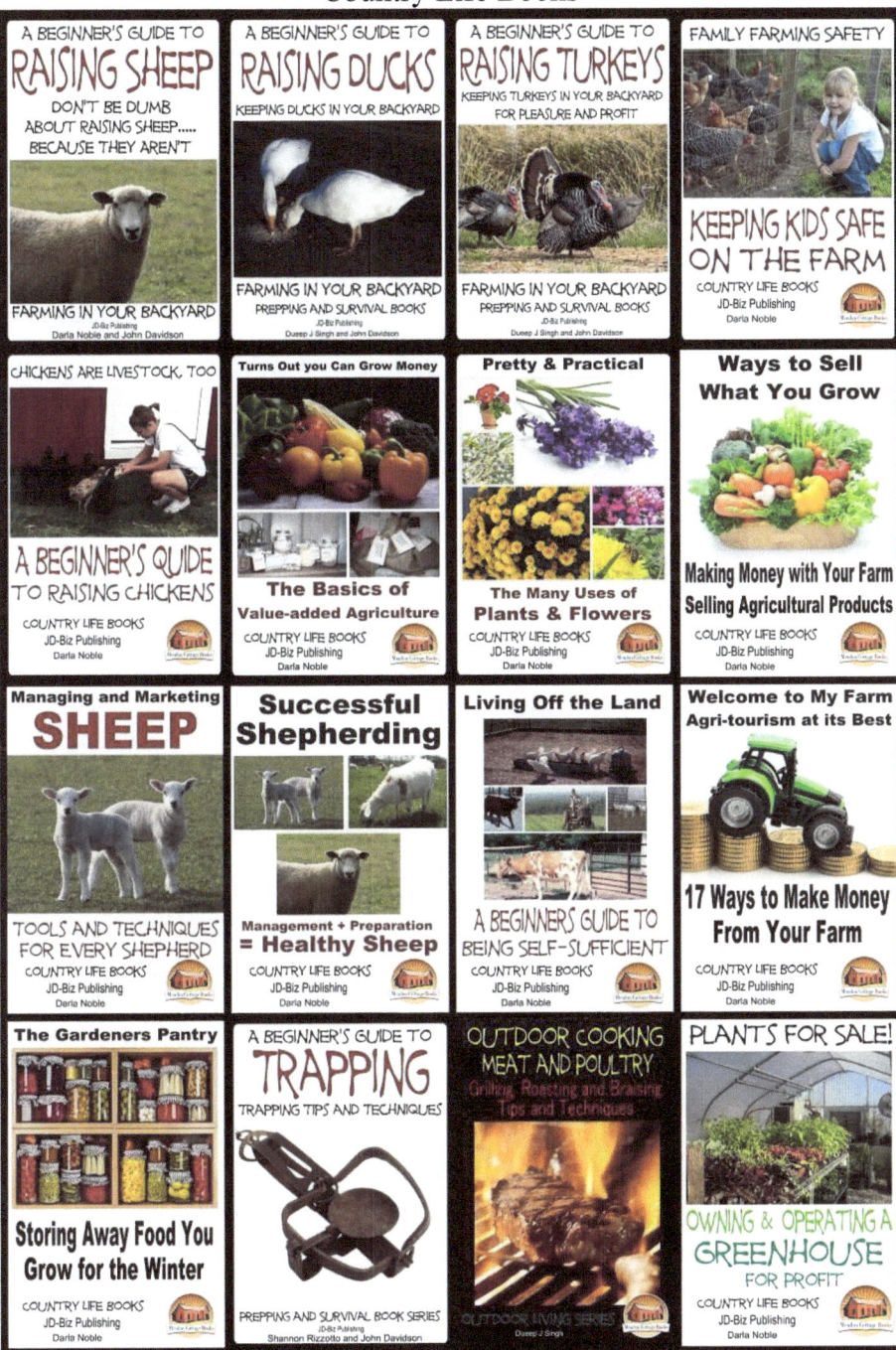

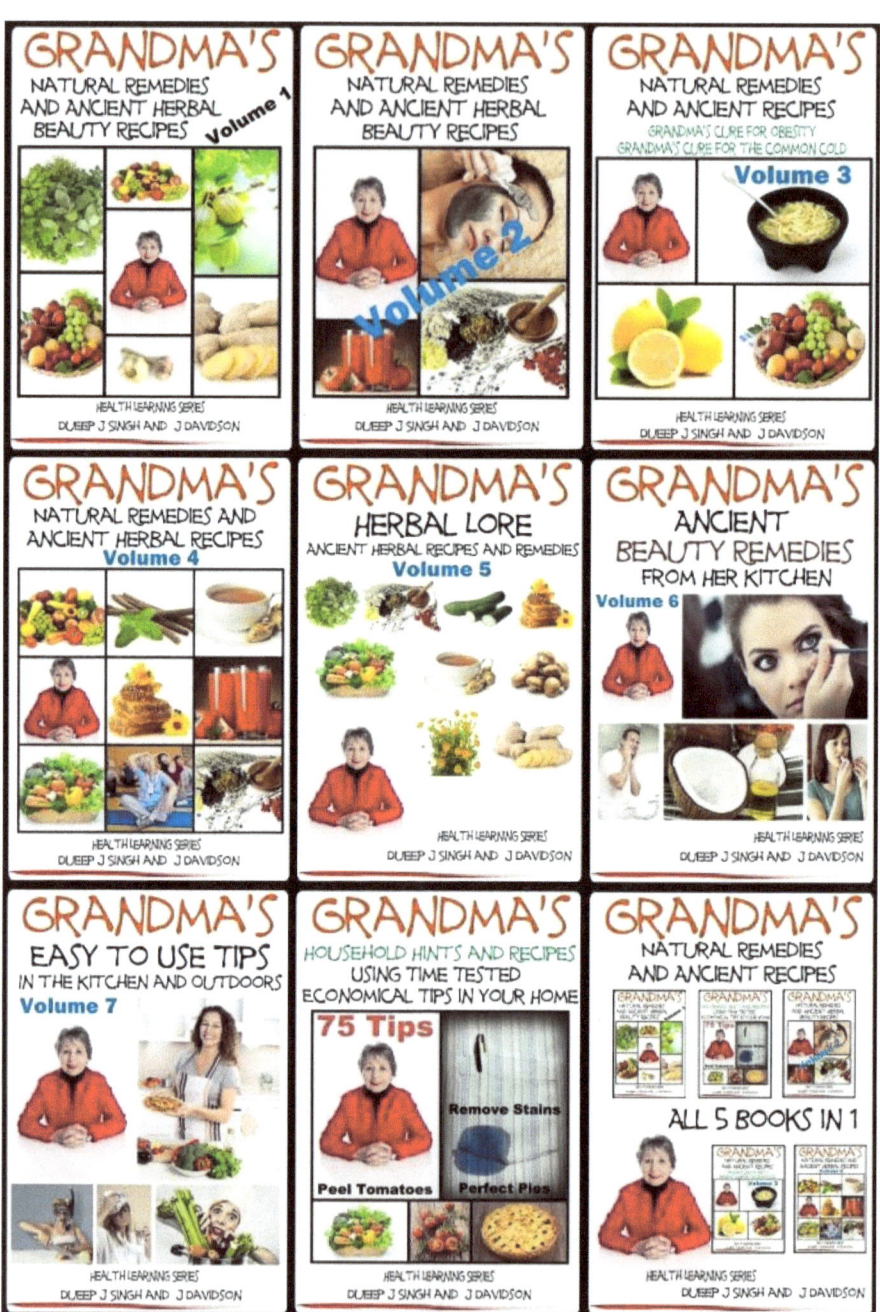

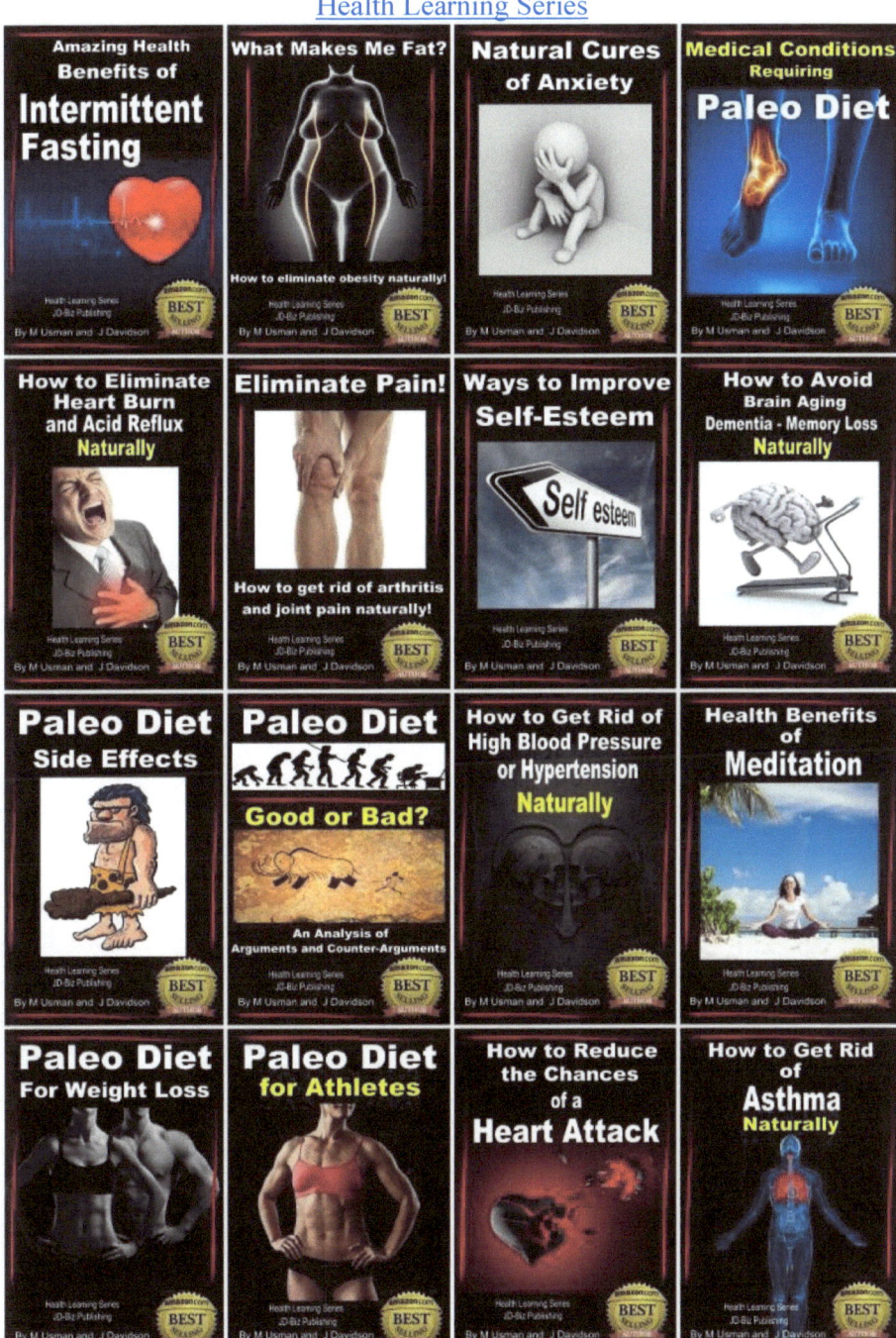

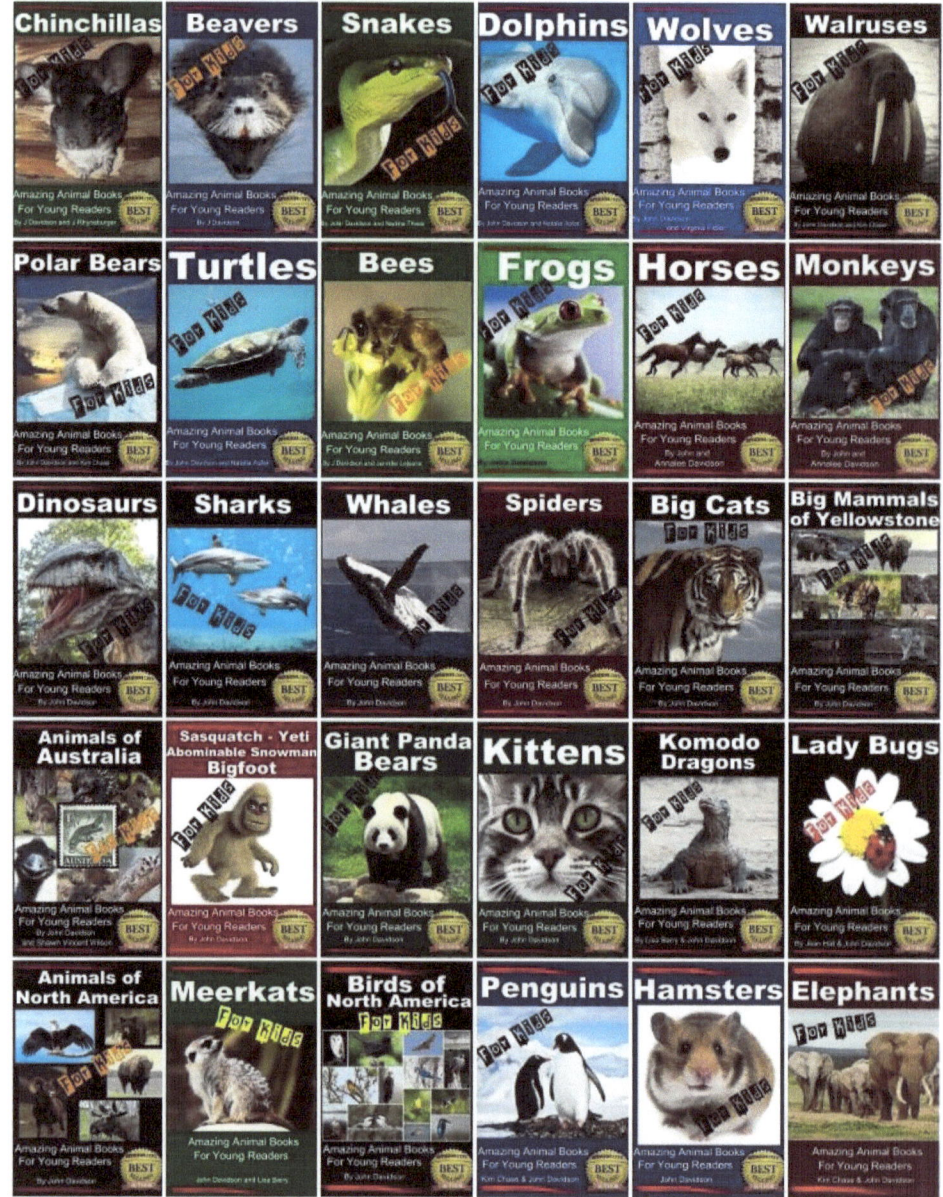

Learn To Draw Series

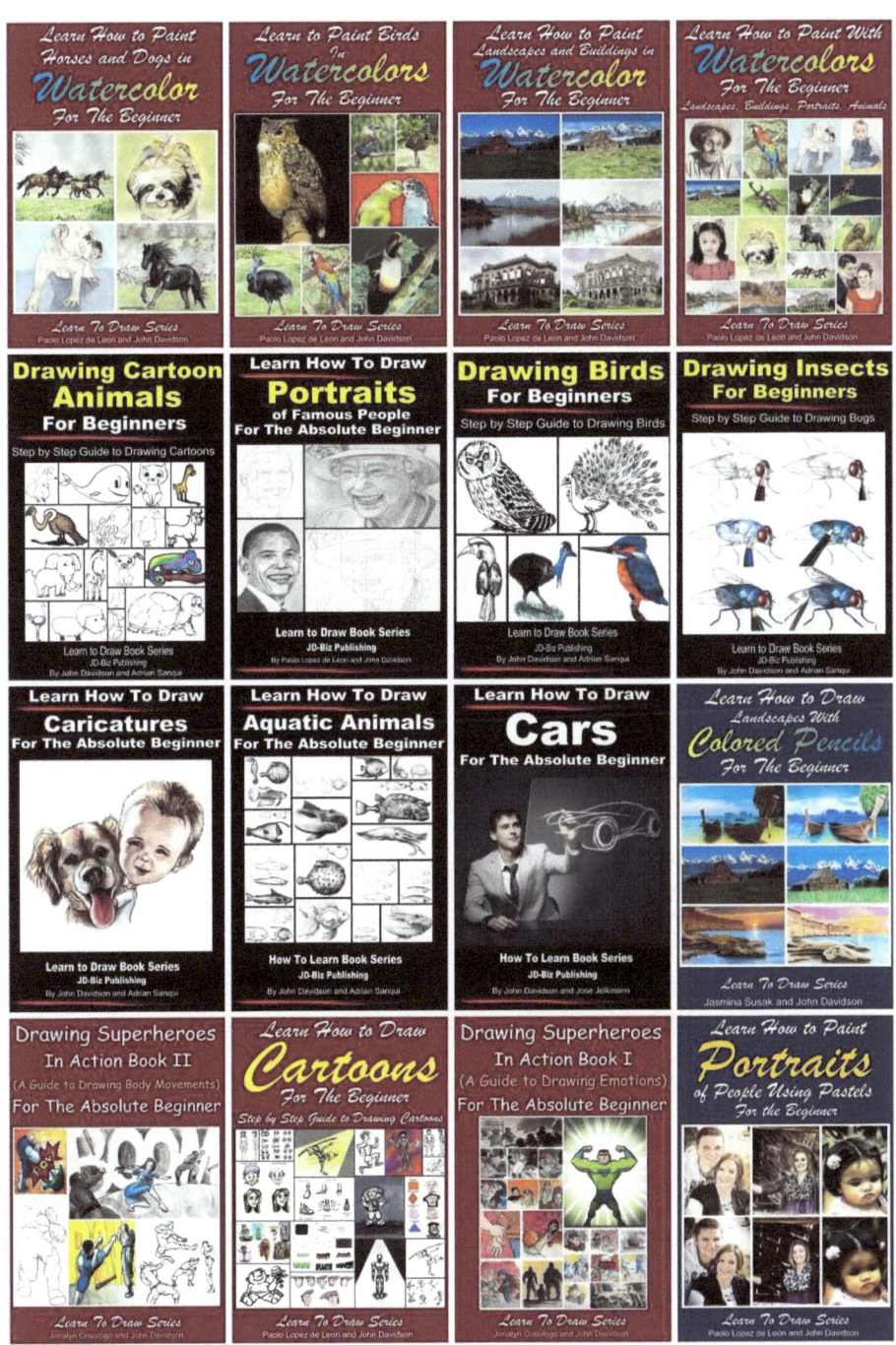

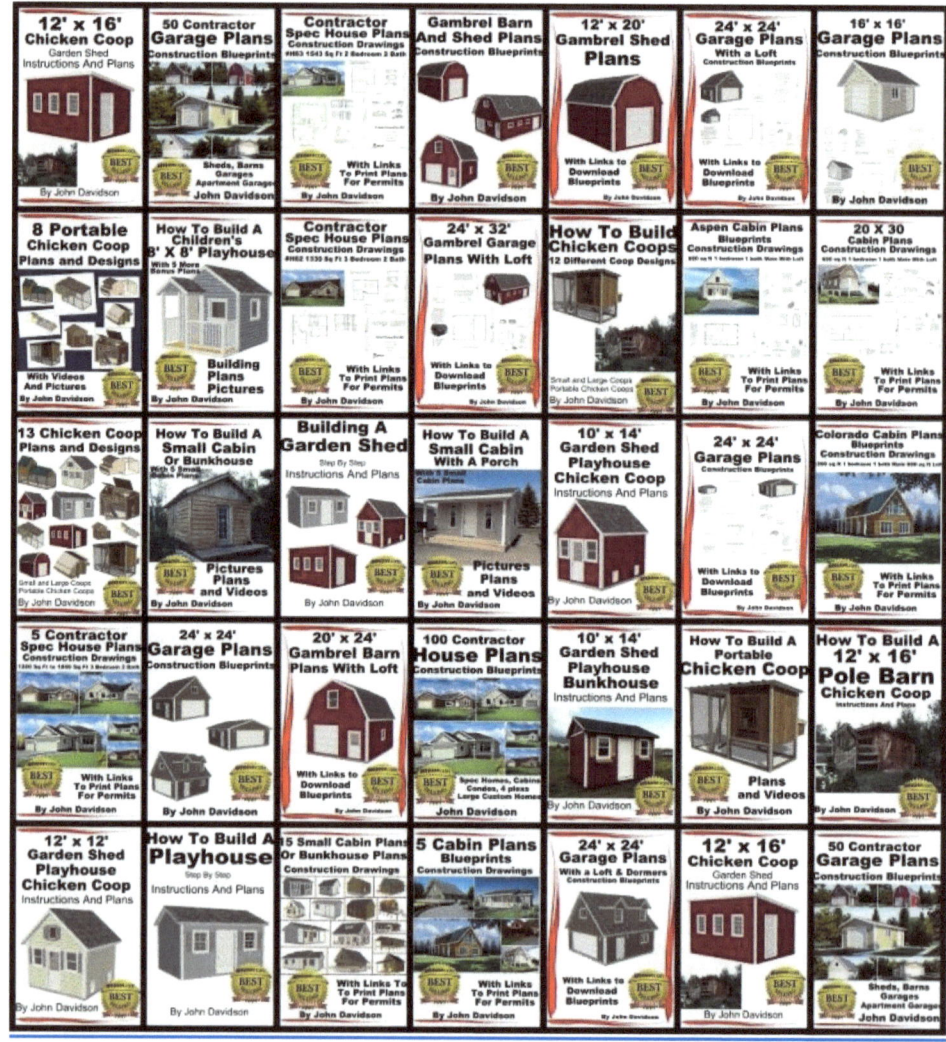

Entrepreneur Book Series

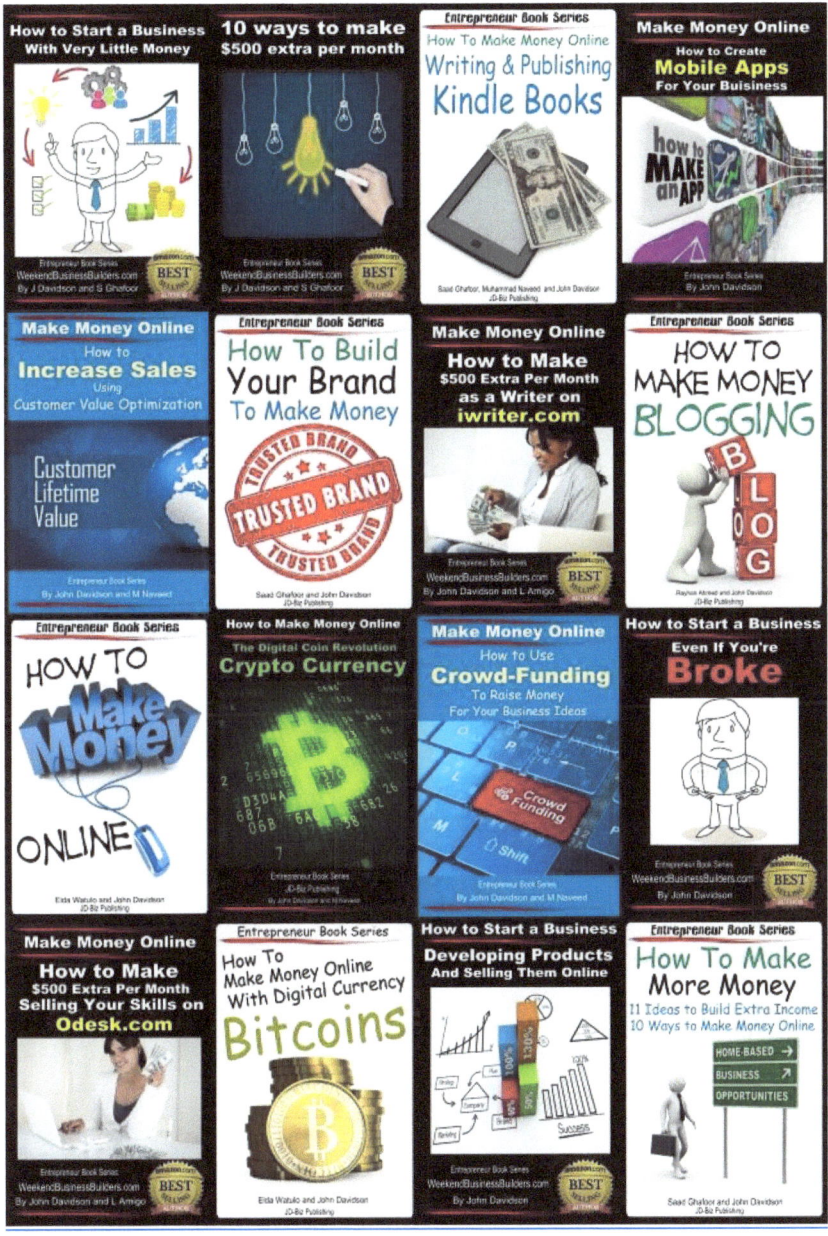

Our books are available at

1. Amazon.com

2. Barnes and Noble

3. Itunes

4. Kobo

5. Smashwords

6. Google Play Books

Publisher

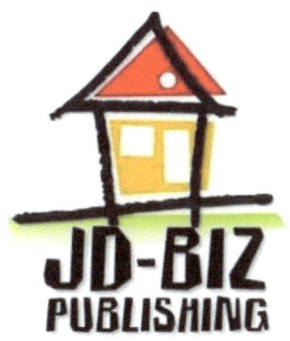

JD-Biz Corp

P O Box 374

Mendon, Utah 84325

http://www.jd-biz.com/

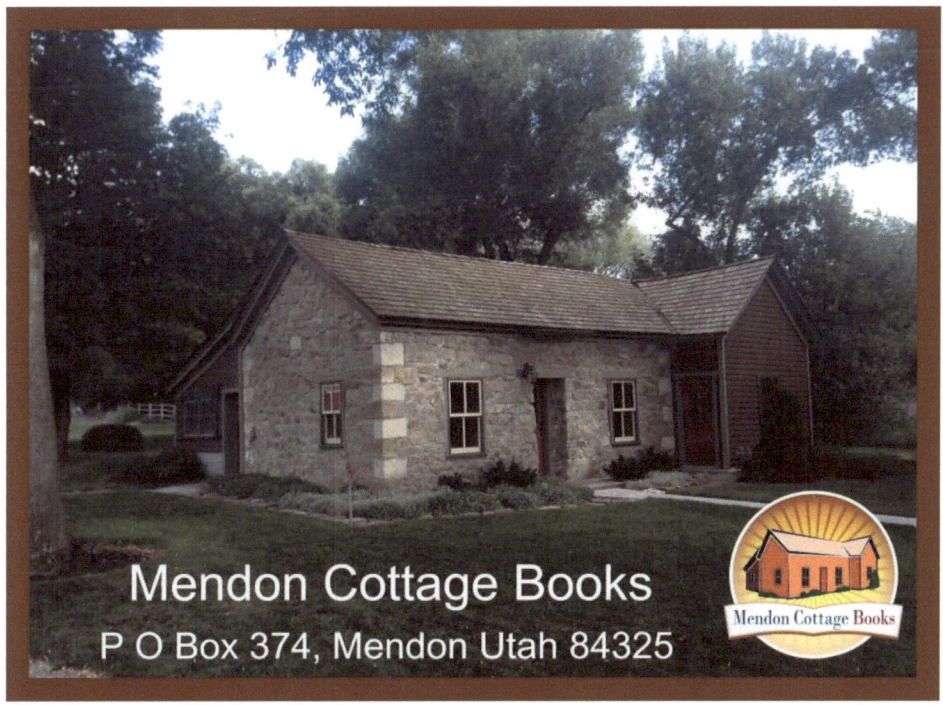

www.ingramcontent.com/pod-product-compliance
Lightning Source LLC
Chambersburg PA
CBHW050836290526
45792CB00001B/417